This journal Belongs

Name: _____

Mobile: _____

E-mail: _____

Age: _____

Weight: _____

Height: _____

Paleo Diet

You've accepted the challenge - Yay! Welcome to 30 Days of Paleo! Here's a way to keep track of your diet. Don't forget that there's a Paleo Journal to help you! which is easily sortable with Nutrition info & Net/Total Carb Counts. You can do it! GOOD LUCK

STARTING WEIGHT:

Day30 WEIGHT:

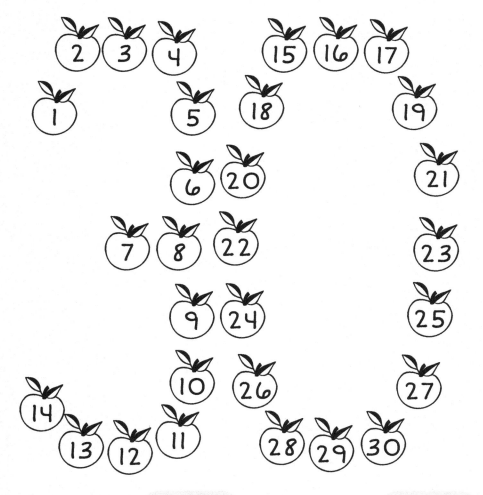

Total weight lost:

Total inches lost:

CONGRATS! YOU DID THAT ! YOU MADE IT!
NOW LET'S DO ANOTHER ROUND OF 60 DAYS OF PALEO!

FIRST OF BODY MEASUREMENTS

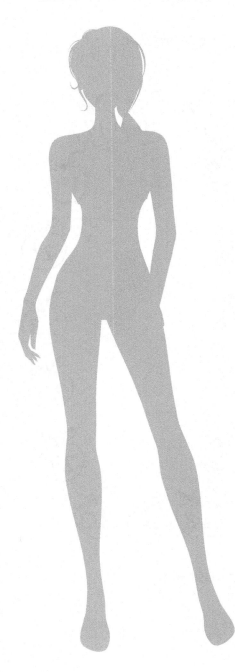

NECK:

Left Arm:

Right Arm:

CHEST:

WAIST:

HIPS:

Left Thigh:

Right Thigh:

Left Calf:

Right Calf:

Weight:

Heart Rate:

Blood Pressure:

END OF MEASUREMENTS

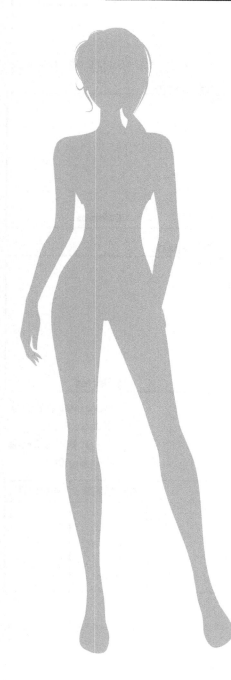

NECK:

Left Arm:

Right Arm:

CHEST:

WAIST:

HIPS:

Left Thigh:

Right Thigh:

Left Calf:

Right Calf:

Weight:

Heart Rate:

Blood Pressure:

Wake Time

Sleep Time

Paleo Food Log

Day 1

DATE:

JAN FEB MAR APR MAY JUN JUL AUG SEP OCT NOV DEC

Breakfast:

Calories:

Lunch:

Calories:

Dinner:

Calories:

Snack:

Calories:

Water Intake

☐ **Vegetables&Fruits**
☐ **Meats&Seafood**
☐ **Eggs, Nuts& Seeds**
☐ **Healthy Oils**

Vitamins

Medicine

🏋 Today's Workout	CALORIES	WEIGHT

Today I feel.....

NOTES

Paleo Food Log

Wake Time

Sleep Time

Day 2

DATE:

JAN FEB MAR APR MAY JUN JUL AUG SEP OCT NOV DEC

Breakfast:

Calories: _____

Lunch:

Calories: _____

Dinner:

Calories: _____

Snack:

Calories: _____

Water Intake

- [ ] Vegetables&Fruits
- [ ] Meats&Seafood
- [ ] Eggs, Nuts& Seeds
- [ ] Healthy Oils

Vitamins _____   Medicine _____

🏋 Today's Workout	CALORIES	WEIGHT

Today I feel.....

NOTES

_____
_____
_____
_____

Wake Time

Sleep Time

Paleo Food Log

| Day 3 |

DATE:

JAN FEB MAR APR MAY JUN JUL AUG SEP OCT NOV DEC

Breakfast:

Calories: _____

Lunch:

Calories: _____

Dinner:

Calories: _____

Snack:

Calories: _____

Water Intake

☐ Vitamins _____   ☐ Medicine _____

☐ Vegetables&Fruits
☐ Meats&Seafood
☐ Eggs, Nuts& Seeds
☐ Healthy Oils

🏋 Today's Workout	CALORIES	WEIGHT

Today I feel.....

NOTES

_____
_____
_____
_____

Wake Time

Sleep Time

Paleo Food Log

Day 4

DATE:

JAN FEB MAR APR MAY JUN JUL AUG SEP OCT NOV DEC

Breakfast:

Calories: _____

Lunch:

Calories: _____

Dinner:

Calories: _____

Snack:

Calories: _____

Water Intake

☐ **Vegetables&Fruits**
☐ **Meats&Seafood**
☐ **Eggs, Nuts& Seeds**
☐ **Healthy Oils**

Vitamins _____   **Medicine** _____

🏋 Today's Workout	CALORIES	WEIGHT

Today I feel.....

NOTES
_____
_____
_____
_____

Wake Time

Sleep Time

Paleo Food Log

Day 5

DATE:

JAN FEB MAR APR MAY JUN JUL AUG SEP OCT NOV DEC

Breakfast:

Calories:

Lunch:

Calories:

Dinner:

Calories:

Snack:

Calories:

Water Intake

Vitamins

Medicine

- [ ] **Vegetables&Fruits**
- [ ] **Meats&Seafood**
- [ ] **Eggs, Nuts& Seeds**
- [ ] **Healthy Oils**

Today's Workout	CALORIES	WEIGHT

Today I feel.....

NOTES

Wake Time

Sleep Time

Paleo Food Log

Day 6

DATE:

JAN FEB MAR APR MAY JUN JUL AUG SEP OCT NOV DEC

Breakfast:

Calories: _____

Lunch:

Calories: _____

Dinner:

Calories: _____

Snack:

Calories: _____

Water Intake

- [ ] Vegetables&Fruits
- [ ] Meats&Seafood
- [ ] Eggs, Nuts& Seeds
- [ ] Healthy Oils

Vitamins _____

Medicine _____

🏋 Today's Workout	CALORIES	WEIGHT

Today I feel.....

NOTES

_____
_____
_____
_____

Wake Time

Sleep Time

Paleo Food Log

Day
7

DATE:

JAN FEB MAR APR MAY JUN JUL AUG SEP OCT NOV DEC

Breakfast:

Calories:

Lunch:

Calories:

Dinner:

Calories:

Snack:

Calories:

Water Intake

Vitamins

Medicine

- Vegetables&Fruits
- Meats&Seafood
- Eggs, Nuts& Seeds
- Healthy Oils

Today's Workout	CALORIES	WEIGHT

Today I feel.....

NOTES

Wake Time 🕐

Sleep Time 🕐

Paleo Food Log

| Day 8 |

DATE:

JAN FEB MAR APR MAY JUN JUL AUG SEP OCT NOV DEC

🍴 **Breakfast:**

Calories: _____

🥄 **Lunch:**

Calories: _____

🍴 **Dinner:**

Calories: _____

🥄 **Snack:**

Calories: _____

Water Intake 🥤🥤🥤🥤🥤🥤🥤🥤

☐ **Vegetables&Fruits**
☐ **Meats&Seafood**
☐ **Eggs, Nuts& Seeds**
☐ **Healthy Oils**

💊 **Vitamins** [_____]   ⚪ **Medicine** [_____]

🏋️ Today's Workout	CALORIES	WEIGHT

Today I feel.....

😊 😠 😆
😓 🥰 😵

NOTES

_____
_____
_____
_____

Wake Time

Sleep Time

Paleo Food Log

Day 9

DATE:

JAN FEB MAR APR MAY JUN JUL AUG SEP OCT NOV DEC

Breakfast:

Calories: _____

Lunch:

Calories: _____

Dinner:

Calories: _____

Snack:

Calories: _____

Water Intake

Vitamins [   ]

Medicine [   ]

- [ ] Vegetables&Fruits
- [ ] Meats&Seafood
- [ ] Eggs, Nuts& Seeds
- [ ] Healthy Oils

🏋 Today's Workout	CALORIES	WEIGHT

Today I feel.....

NOTES

_____

_____

_____

_____

Wake Time

Paleo Food Log

Day 10

Sleep Time

DATE:

Breakfast:

Calories:

Lunch:

Calories:

Dinner:

Calories:

Snack:

Calories:

Water Intake

☐ **Vegetables&Fruits**
☐ **Meats&Seafood**
☐ **Eggs, Nuts& Seeds**
☐ **Healthy Oils**

Vitamins [   ]   **Medicine** [   ]

🏋 Today's Workout	CALORIES	WEIGHT

Today I feel.....

NOTES

_____
_____
_____
_____

Wake Time 🕐

Paleo Food Log

Day 11

Sleep Time 🕐

DATE:

JAN FEB MAR APR MAY JUN JUL AUG SEP OCT NOV DEC

🍽 Breakfast:

Calories: _____

🍽 Lunch:

Calories: _____

🍽 Dinner:

Calories: _____

🍽 Snack:

Calories: _____

Water Intake 🥤🥤🥤🥤🥤🥤🥤🥤🥤🥤

☐ **Vegetables&Fruits**
☐ **Meats&Seafood**
☐ **Eggs, Nuts& Seeds**
☐ **Healthy Oils**

💊 **Vitamins** [_____]   ⬤ **Medicine** [_____]

🏋 Today's Workout	CALORIES	WEIGHT

Today I feel.....

😊 😠 😏

🥱 😍 😴

NOTES

_____
_____
_____
_____

Wake Time

Sleep Time

Paleo Food Log

Day 12

DATE:

JAN FEB MAR APR MAY JUN JUL AUG SEP OCT NOV DEC

Breakfast:

Calories: _____

Lunch:

Calories: _____

Dinner:

Calories: _____

Snack:

Calories: _____

Water Intake

- [ ] Vegetables&Fruits
- [ ] Meats&Seafood
- [ ] Eggs, Nuts& Seeds
- [ ] Healthy Oils

Vitamins _____   **Medicine** _____

🏋 Today's Workout	CALORIES	WEIGHT

Today I feel.....

NOTES

_____
_____
_____
_____

Wake Time

Sleep Time

Paleo Food Log

Day 13

DATE:

JAN FEB MAR APR MAY JUN JUL AUG SEP OCT NOV DEC

Breakfast:

Calories: _____

Lunch:

Calories: _____

Dinner:

Calories: _____

Snack:

Calories: _____

Water Intake

☐ **Vegetables&Fruits**
☐ **Meats&Seafood**
☐ **Eggs, Nuts& Seeds**
☐ **Healthy Oils**

Vitamins _____   **Medicine** _____

🏋 Today's Workout	CALORIES	WEIGHT

Today I feel.....

NOTES

_____
_____
_____
_____

Wake Time

Sleep Time

Paleo Food Log

Day 14

DATE:

JAN FEB MAR APR MAY JUN JUL AUG SEP OCT NOV DEC

Breakfast:

Calories: _____

Lunch:

Calories: _____

Dinner:

Calories: _____

Snack:

Calories: _____

Water Intake

☐ **Vegetables&Fruits**
☐ **Meats&Seafood**
☐ **Eggs, Nuts& Seeds**
☐ **Healthy Oils**

🔹 **Vitamins** _____   ⬤ **Medicine** _____

⚡ Today's Workout	CALORIES	WEIGHT

Today I feel.....

NOTES
_____
_____
_____
_____

Wake Time

Sleep Time

Paleo Food Log

Day 15

DATE:

JAN FEB MAR APR MAY JUN JUL AUG SEP OCT NOV DEC

Breakfast:

Calories: _____

Lunch:

Calories: _____

Dinner:

Calories: _____

Snack:

Calories: _____

Water Intake

Vitamins [ ]

Medicine [ ]

- [ ] Vegetables&Fruits
- [ ] Meats&Seafood
- [ ] Eggs, Nuts& Seeds
- [ ] Healthy Oils

💪 Today's Workout	CALORIES	WEIGHT

Today I feel.....

NOTES

_____
_____
_____
_____

Wake Time 🕐

Sleep Time 🕐

Paleo Food Log

| Day 16 |

DATE:

JAN FEB MAR APR MAY JUN JUL AUG SEP OCT NOV DEC

🍽 Breakfast:

Calories: _____

🍽 Lunch:

Calories: _____

🍽 Dinner:

Calories: _____

🍽 Snack:

Calories: _____

Water Intake 🥤🥤🥤🥤🥤🥤🥤🥤🥤🥤

🔲 **Vegetables&Fruits**
🔲 **Meats&Seafood**
🔲 **Eggs, Nuts& Seeds**
🔲 **Healthy Oils**

🔹 **Vitamins** _____   ⚪ **Medicine** _____

🏋 Today's Workout	CALORIES	WEIGHT

Today I feel.....

😊 😠 😏
☕ 😍 😴

NOTES

_____
_____
_____
_____

Wake Time

Sleep Time

Paleo Food Log

Day 17

DATE:

JAN FEB MAR APR MAY JUN JUL AUG SEP OCT NOV DEC

Breakfast:

Calories: _____

Lunch:

Calories: _____

Dinner:

Calories: _____

Snack:

Calories: _____

Water Intake

☐ **Vegetables&Fruits**
☐ **Meats&Seafood**
☐ **Eggs, Nuts& Seeds**
☐ **Healthy Oils**

Vitamins [   ]   **Medicine** [   ]

🏋 Today's Workout	CALORIES	WEIGHT

Today I feel.....

NOTES

_____
_____
_____
_____

Wake Time

Sleep Time

Paleo Food Log

Day 18

DATE:

JAN FEB MAR APR MAY JUN JUL AUG SEP OCT NOV DEC

Breakfast:

Calories: _____

Lunch:

Calories: _____

Dinner:

Calories: _____

Snack:

Calories: _____

Water Intake

Vitamins _____   **Medicine** _____

☐ **Vegetables&Fruits**
☐ **Meats&Seafood**
☐ **Eggs, Nuts& Seeds**
☐ **Healthy Oils**

Today's Workout	CALORIES	WEIGHT

Today I feel.....

NOTES

_____
_____
_____
_____

Wake Time

Sleep Time

Paleo Food Log

Day 19

DATE:

JAN FEB MAR APR MAY JUN JUL AUG SEP OCT NOV DEC

Breakfast:

Calories: _____

Lunch:

Calories: _____

Dinner:

Calories: _____

Snack:

Calories: _____

Water Intake

☐ **Vegetables&Fruits**
☐ **Meats&Seafood**
☐ **Eggs, Nuts& Seeds**
☐ **Healthy Oils**

🖊 **Vitamins** _____   ⬤ **Medicine** _____

🏋 Today's Workout	CALORIES	WEIGHT

Today I feel.....

NOTES
_____
_____
_____
_____

Paleo Food Log

Day 20

Wake Time

Sleep Time

DATE:

JAN FEB MAR APR MAY JUN JUL AUG SEP OCT NOV DEC

Breakfast:

Calories: _____

Lunch:

Calories: _____

Dinner:

Calories: _____

Snack:

Calories: _____

Water Intake

Vitamins [   ]

Medicine [   ]

- [ ] Vegetables&Fruits
- [ ] Meats&Seafood
- [ ] Eggs, Nuts& Seeds
- [ ] Healthy Oils

Today's Workout	CALORIES	WEIGHT

Today I feel.....

NOTES

_____
_____
_____
_____

Wake Time 🕐

Sleep Time 🕐

Paleo Food Log

DATE:

JAN FEB MAR APR MAY JUN JUL AUG SEP OCT NOV DEC

🍴 **Breakfast:**

Calories: _____

🍴 **Lunch:**

Calories: _____

🍴 **Dinner:**

Calories: _____

🍴 **Snack:**

Calories: _____

Water Intake 🥤🥤🥤🥤🥤🥤🥤🥤🥤🥤

💊 **Vitamins** [_____]   ⬤ **Medicine** [_____]

☐ **Vegetables&Fruits**
☐ **Meats&Seafood**
☐ **Eggs, Nuts& Seeds**
☐ **Healthy Oils**

🏋️ Today's Workout	CALORIES	WEIGHT

Today I feel.....

😊 😠 😆
😓 😍 😋

NOTES

_____
_____
_____
_____

Wake Time

Sleep Time

Paleo Food Log

Day 22

DATE:

JAN FEB MAR APR MAY JUN JUL AUG SEP OCT NOV DEC

Breakfast:

Calories: _____

Lunch:

Calories: _____

Dinner:

Calories: _____

Snack:

Calories: _____

Water Intake

Vitamins _____

Medicine _____

- [ ] Vegetables&Fruits
- [ ] Meats&Seafood
- [ ] Eggs, Nuts& Seeds
- [ ] Healthy Oils

🏋 Today's Workout	CALORIES	WEIGHT

Today I feel.....

NOTES

_____
_____
_____
_____

Wake Time

Sleep Time

Paleo Food Log

DATE:

JAN FEB MAR APR MAY JUN JUL AUG SEP OCT NOV DEC

Breakfast:

Calories: _____

Lunch:

Calories: _____

Dinner:

Calories: _____

Snack:

Calories: _____

Water Intake

Vitamins [_____]   **Medicine** [_____]

- [ ] **Vegetables&Fruits**
- [ ] **Meats&Seafood**
- [ ] **Eggs, Nuts& Seeds**
- [ ] **Healthy Oils**

Today's Workout	CALORIES	WEIGHT

Today I feel.....

NOTES

_____
_____
_____
_____

Wake Time

Sleep Time

Paleo Food Log

Day 24

DATE:

JAN FEB MAR APR MAY JUN JUL AUG SEP OCT NOV DEC

Breakfast:

Calories: _____

Lunch:

Calories: _____

Dinner:

Calories: _____

Snack:

Calories: _____

Water Intake

Vitamins _____

Medicine _____

- Vegetables&Fruits
- Meats&Seafood
- Eggs, Nuts& Seeds
- Healthy Oils

🏋 Today's Workout	CALORIES	WEIGHT

Today I feel.....

NOTES

_____
_____
_____
_____

Paleo Food Log

Day 25

Wake Time

Sleep Time

DATE:

Breakfast:

Calories: _____

Lunch:

Calories: _____

Dinner:

Calories: _____

Snack:

Calories: _____

Water Intake

- [ ] Vegetables&Fruits
- [ ] Meats&Seafood
- [ ] Eggs, Nuts& Seeds
- [ ] Healthy Oils

Vitamins _____

Medicine _____

🏋️ Today's Workout	CALORIES	WEIGHT

Today I feel.....

NOTES

_____
_____
_____
_____

Paleo Food Log

Day 26

Wake Time

Sleep Time

DATE:

JAN FEB MAR APR MAY JUN JUL AUG SEP OCT NOV DEC

Breakfast:

Calories:

Lunch:

Calories:

Dinner:

Calories:

Snack:

Calories:

Water Intake

- [ ] Vegetables&Fruits
- [ ] Meats&Seafood
- [ ] Eggs, Nuts& Seeds
- [ ] Healthy Oils

Vitamins

Medicine

🏋 Today's Workout	CALORIES	WEIGHT

Today I feel.....

NOTES

Wake Time ⏰

Sleep Time ⏰

Paleo Food Log

Day 27

DATE:

JAN FEB MAR APR MAY JUN JUL AUG SEP OCT NOV DEC

🍴 **Breakfast:**

Calories: _____

🍴 **Lunch:**

Calories: _____

🍴 **Dinner:**

Calories: _____

🍴 **Snack:**

Calories: _____

Water Intake 🥤🥤🥤🥤🥤🥤🥤🥤🥤🥤

🔲 Vegetables&Fruits
🔲 Meats&Seafood
🔲 Eggs, Nuts& Seeds
🔲 Healthy Oils

💊 **Vitamins** _____   ⚪ **Medicine** _____

🏋️ Today's Workout	CALORIES	WEIGHT

Today I feel.....

😊 😠 😆
😋 😍 😴

NOTES

_____
_____
_____
_____

Wake Time

Sleep Time

Paleo Food Log

Day 28

DATE:

JAN FEB MAR APR MAY JUN JUL AUG SEP OCT NOV DEC

Breakfast:

Calories:

Lunch:

Calories:

Dinner:

Calories:

Snack:

Calories:

Water Intake

Vitamins

Medicine

- [ ] **Vegetables&Fruits**
- [ ] **Meats&Seafood**
- [ ] **Eggs, Nuts& Seeds**
- [ ] **Healthy Oils**

🏋 Today's Workout	CALORIES	WEIGHT

Today I feel.....

NOTES

Wake Time

Sleep Time

Paleo Food Log

Day 29

DATE:

JAN FEB MAR APR MAY JUN JUL AUG SEP OCT NOV DEC

Breakfast:

Calories: ________

Lunch:

Calories: ________

Dinner:

Calories: ________

Snack:

Calories: ________

Water Intake

Vitamins

Medicine

- [ ] Vegetables&Fruits
- [ ] Meats&Seafood
- [ ] Eggs, Nuts& Seeds
- [ ] Healthy Oils

Today's Workout	CALORIES	WEIGHT

Today I feel.....

NOTES

Wake Time

Sleep Time

Paleo Food Log

| Day 30 |

DATE:

JAN FEB MAR APR MAY JUN JUL AUG SEP OCT NOV DEC

Breakfast:

Calories: _____

Lunch:

Calories: _____

Dinner:

Calories: _____

Snack:

Calories: _____

Water Intake

☐ **Vegetables&Fruits**
☐ **Meats&Seafood**
☐ **Eggs, Nuts& Seeds**
☐ **Healthy Oils**

🔹 **Vitamins** [_____]   🔘 **Medicine** [_____]

🏋️ Today's Workout	CALORIES	WEIGHT

Today I feel.....

NOTES

_____
_____
_____
_____

CONGRATS! YOU DID THAT ! YOU MADE IT!

Made in the USA
Las Vegas, NV
29 November 2022

60656058R00056